I0427900

50 Natural Masks and Scrubs

Beautify Yourself Right at Home with Homemade Masks and Scrubs

Disclaimer

No part of this book can be transmitted or reproduced in any form including print, electronic, photocopying, scanning, mechanical or recording without the author's permission.

The author has tried to be an authentic source of the information provided in this report. However, the author does not oppose the additional information available over the internet. The information included in this book cannot be compared with information of the same provided in other books. All readers can seek further help through additional sources of information.

Ignoring any of the guidelines for the tips or not following each step of the preparation method of the recipes may not give you the exact result. Therefore, the author is not responsible for such negligence.

What This EBook Contains

In this world of pollution and harmful bacteria, taking care of yourself–in terms of both physical and mental health–has become a must. But with the rise in cost of skincare products, it becomes literally impossible for 80% of the population to pamper and take care of themselves. This is the reason why more and more people are opting for natural, homemade products in order to achieve a healthy and glowing self.

The best part about using organic, homemade skincare products is that not only are they extremely inexpensive, they are also free from all chemicals and hazardous substances. If you too have been looking for scrub and masks recipes that will make your skin shiny and soft, try going through this entire eBook.

This eBook will tell you all you need to know about:

a) Why skincare is important

b) What are scrubs and masks?

c) Recipes for 25 scrubs and 25 masks

d) How you can make them using easy-to-find ingredients right at home

e) What are the benefits of the recipes and the ingredients used?

f) Simple process of making and storing the recipes

g) Some tips and alternative ingredients you can use

By the time you have completed reading this eBook, you will no longer feel the need to buy scrubs and masks from the store. You can even gift wrap them and give them to your loved ones. Trust us, they will love the effort you have put in making your very own skincare product for them!

So without further talk, let us learn how you can whip up your own masks and scrubs, right in your very own kitchen!

Contents

Introduction

Keeping your skin fresh, hydrated and supple has become more difficult now than it was before. This has happened mainly because of the fact that the environment seems to be getting dirtier by the second. Smoke, chemical pollutants and the harsh rays of sun leave the skin stripped of all healthy nutrients and natural beauty. And this is why you should take extra care so that you can look your best without the use of multiple cosmetics.

Scrubs

A scrub, be it for face, hands, feet or body, is an excellent remedy for dead and damaged skin. It works in a way that, even though the deadened skin is removed, your skin is not harmed in any way. Unlike chemical-based commercial products that can harm your face or body, natural homemade scrubs are completely safe.

The great thing about using scrubs is that their regular use leaves the skin smooth and even-toned. The skin remains fresh and dewy, giving you skin like that of a baby. It is also great for the complete removal of makeup. This of course does not mean that you should overdo the use. Using a scrub twice a week is enough. Too much of anything can be harmful, so do not irritate your skin by using a scrub every single day.

Masks

Like scrubs, masks work just as efficiently. It not only leaves your skin squeaky clean, it also smoothes, tones, firms up and revitalizes your skin. They are also great for the repair of damaged skin tissues. But the best thing about masks is that they are very relaxing. Imagine coming back from a hard day of work, applying a soothing mask on your face and relaxing for 15-20 minutes. The mask will leave you feeling calm and serene. It will also freshen up your face within no time.

So want to know how you can get all these skincare products without spending hundreds of dollars? Make them right at home! Here are 50 recipes for you.

25 Effective Scrubs

The 25 recipes given below are effective for most skin kinds. It is recommended that you try the scrub on a small patch of skin before using it, so that you can be clear about whether or not the product even suits you. If you are allergic to any of the ingredients, do not use them.

If you have some kind of skin condition, be sure to ask a medical health professional before using anything. These scrubs are mild enough to be used on sensitive skin too.

5 Body Scrubs

Body scrubs are great for people of all ages. They are especially beneficial during winters. By removing dead skin, they give your body a healthy glow and also get you out of the misery of skin peeling off. You can change some of the ingredients to suit your skin type and needs, but it is recommended that you follow the recipes as it is.

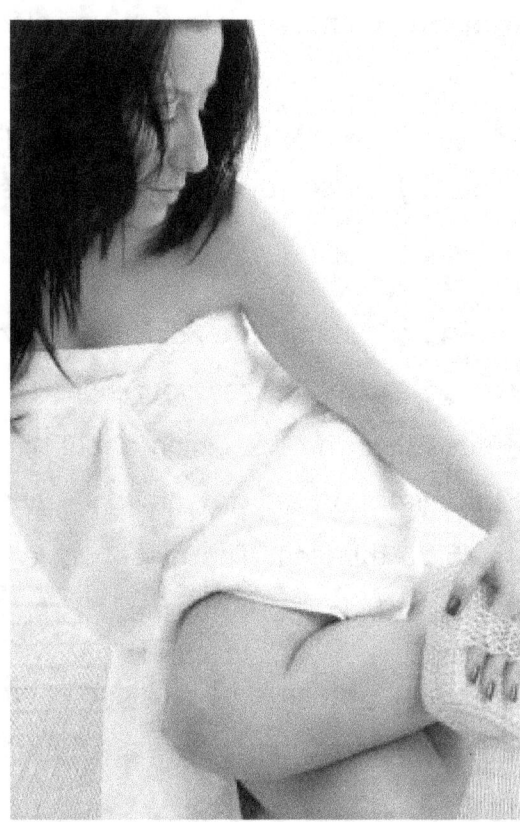

Cinnamony Sweet Scrub

Cinnamon is one of the best anti-bacterial herbs ever. It also smells divine. If you are looking for sugary goodness, then this scrub is the one for you!

Ingredients

3 drops of cinnamon essential oil

½ cup of white or brown sugar ¼ cup of coconut oil

½ cup of raw cane sugar

½ tsp. of vanilla extract

Pinch of cinnamon

Process

Combine all the ingredients together except for the coconut oil. Then slowly add the base oil and keep mixing until well combined. Once you get a scrub-like texture, store in a tightly-lidded glass bottle. All you have to do is make sure that your body is a little wet, then apply the scrub all over. Rub lightly and then wash off. You will feel your skin softening over time.

1. Almond Oil Scrub

Almond oil is great as a softener, as well as moisturizer. Since it is not too dense, it makes the skin supple and smooth. Here is how you can incorporate it in a scrub:

Ingredients

½ cup almond oil

1 cup brown or white sugar (granulated)

5 vitamin E capsules

5 drops of tea tree essential oil

5 drops of lemon essential oil

Process

Mix almond oil, sugar and essential oils. Break the vitamin E capsules and pour the oil in. Then combine the ingredients together and store in a jar. When using, wet your body and gently massage the scrub on, starting from the neck. Wash off with warm water.

2. Salty Rosemary Scrub

Imagine rubbing something on your body that smells like rosemary! Can it get any better? It can when there is salt mixed in it. Salt is one of the best exfoliants there is!

Ingredients

2 tbsp. of crushed rosemary leaves

¼ cup olive oil

½ cup of sea salt or kosher salt

1 tbsp. of lavender extract

Process

Simply mix all the ingredients together and store in a glass or Mason jar. Use twice a week before taking a bath. Make sure you scrub gently, as rubbing vigorously can irritate the skin. Once you have massaged the scrub on your body, leave on for 5 minutes and then wash off.

3. Bye to Cellulite Scrub

Cellulite can be one of the worst things that can happen to your body. It does not hurt so much as it looks wrinkly. Caffeine is said to be the best remedy for this problem, because it promotes proper circulation and helps in clearing away the dead skin.

Ingredients

½ cup of brown sugar

1/4 cup of sea salt

½ cup of coffee

¼ cup of coconut oil

Process

Mix the dry ingredients first and then add in the coconut oil. Mix until combined and then use. When in the bath, massage the scrub on your skin in circular motions and then rinse off with warm water. Make sure you only apply it to affected areas.

4. Minty Scrub

One of the greatest scrubs is one that contains lemon and mint, which is this scrub. It is easy to make and good enough to eat!

Ingredients

½ cup of white granulated sugar

2 tbsp. of spearmint essential oil

¼ cup of grape seed oil

1 tbsp. of fresh lemon juice

Process

Thoroughly combine all the ingredients and apply to wet body. Massage well and then rinse off. Make sure you get it all off. The minty, lemony smell will linger throughout the day, giving you a fresh, sense-stimulating scent.

5 Face Scrubs

Face scrubs are wonderful because they give your face a shine that nothing else can. Try making your very own and see which ones suit your skin type.

5. Oatmeal Scrub

This oatmeal scrub is great for all year round, but works especially well for winters. Make sure you are not allergic to any ingredients before trying it out.

Ingredients

1 cup whole oats (grind them in a food processor to a fine powder)

2 tbsp. of whole milk

1 egg white

A few drops of lavender essential oil

1 tbsp. of brown sugar

1 tsp. of olive oil

Process

Mix all the ingredients well and apply to slightly wet face. Massage thoroughly and leave on for 2-3 minutes. Dip a clean washcloth in warm water and rinse your face clean. Then splash cold water on face to close off all the pores.

6. Choffee Scrub

Coffee and dark chocolate are both wonderful for your face. They brighten the skin and leave it smooth and blemish free. Try this scrub for some amazing results.

Ingredients

½ cup cocoa powder (of dark chocolate)

½ cup finely ground coffee

¼ cup honey

¼ cup sweet almond oil

Process

Combine all the ingredients until a paste is formed and apply gently to the skin. Rub lightly so that all the dead skin comes off. Wash off the scrub with warm water and then put a warm wash cloth on face for a while. Take that off and rub an ice cube lightly all over your face. You will notice an immediate glow to your skin.

7. Green Tea Scrub

Green tea isn't only great for your digestive system, it is also wonderful for your skin. You can drink it and apply it to the face for mind blowing results. Try this green tea scrub and see the effects yourself.

<u>Ingredients</u>

1 ½ tsp. loose green tea leaves

1 cup boiling water

1 tbsp. of white granulated sugar

1 tsp. lemon juice

3 drops rose essential oil

<u>Process</u>

Steep green tea leaves in the boiling water and then strain. Take 3 tbsp. of the tea in a separate bowl, add in the rest of the ingredients and mix well. This is your scrub. Apply to face and massage in circular motion. Rinse off with tap water and pat your face dry.

8. Almond Meal Essential Scrub

Almond meal works just as well as oatmeal. It is great for oily skin. If you have that, this scrub is the one for you.

Ingredients

½ cup plain almonds

½ cup almond oil

A few drops of your favorite essential oil

Process

To make almond meal, simply pulse the almond in a food processor until a rough, grainy texture is obtained. Mix both the oils to this meal and combine well. Apply to face and rub in upward motion. Leave on for 3 minutes and then wash off with warm water. Then splash cold water on face to close off the pores.

9. Peachy Honey Scrub

Peaches work well as an exfoliant, since they contain alpha hydroxyl acid. They will make your skin clearer and smoother. Add honey to the scrub and you have something of a wonder cure for listless skin. Here is how you can make it:

Ingredients

1 ripe, organic peach

½ tbsp. raw honey

1 tbsp. brown sugar

½ tbsp. almond oil

A few drops of tea tree essential oil

Process

Blend the peach in the food processor with some water. Warm up the honey and add it to the pureed peach. Also add the brown sugar, almond oil, tea tree essential oil and mix well. Massage on face and wash off with warm water.

5 Hand Scrubs

Your facial skin is not the only thing that needs to be taken care of. Hand and foot care is just as, if not more, important. The reason why you need to take more care of your hands is that they are used the most for work and all other purposes. Therefore, they demand that we pamper them as much as possible. Below are 5 scrubs to make your hands soft, supple and alive!

10.   Coconut Honey Scrub

This scrub is so good you are going to want to eat it! But please don't, as it is food for hands and not the tummy. Here is how you can make it:

Ingredients

2 tbsp. of raw honey

1 tbsp. of coconut oil

¼ cup organic sugar

¼ cup sea salt

1 tbsp. lemon juice

A few drops of peppermint essential oil

Process

Blend salt, sugar and lemon to the point where it turns to crumbs. Add in honey, coconut oil and essential oil and mix well. Store in a glass jar and use when needed. All you would have to do is dampen your hands and rub it on both hands well. Wash off after 2-3 minutes.

11.   Lemony Scrub

Lemons are quite literally a miracle in small size. They are great for your body, face, hands and even hair! Combine the lemon with hone and you get something that is unrivalled by any commercially produced skincare product.

Ingredients

2 tbsp. lemon juice Some zest of the lemon

4 tbsp of sugar

Olive oil as per need

A few drops of vanilla essence

Process

Mix together all the ingredients and store in the fridge. When needed, take out the scrub, take a dollop on hand and rub gently on both hands. Do this massage for 30 seconds. Rinse with a warm washcloth and then wash off with cool water.

12.   Brown Scrub

Almond oil is great for the hair, raw almonds are efficient memory boosters and almond meal is just the thing your hands begging for. Add honey to this paste you get a scrub that is not just wonderful for you; it is also a great Christmas present!

Ingredients

¼ cup almond meal

2 tbsp. honey

¼ cup brown sugar

3 tbsp. almond oil (sweet)

2 tbsp. tea tree essential oil

Process

Take a glass jar and put all the ingredients in it. Mix well and cover it until needed. When you want to use it, take it out of the fridge and keep it at room temperature for at least 20 minutes. Then dampen your hands and massage gently. Wash off. You won't have a need for a manicure once you start using this!

13.   Lavender Hand Scrub

Want to make your hands glow and smell delicious? Try this scrub for amazing results.

Ingredients

¼ cup white granulated sugar

3 tbsp. of dried lavender

½ tsp. of jojoba oil

Few drops of lavender essential oil

Process

Crush lavender and sugar in a bowl until the lavender starts breaking apart. Add in oils and use as needed. Rub gently on hands for 30 seconds and then rinse off with cool water. Your hands will feel revitalized again!

14. Eucalyptus Sugar Scrub

The best thing about this scrub is that it will leave you with super soft and clean hands. What's more, the enticing smell is bound to turn heads wherever you go. Here is how you can make it.

Ingredients

1 cup white granulated sugar

1 cup raw sugar

1 tbsp. liquid lecithin

1 tsp. vitamin E

1 cup almond or olive oil

Few drops of eucalyptus essential oil

Some lemongrass

Process

Combine all the ingredients together and store in a glass jar. When needed, put some on hands and rub well. Wash off and see the results.

5 Feet Scrubs

Just like your hands, feet also need scrubbing so that dirt and dead skin can be removed and you can have heels that you can show off in strappy sandals. Here are 5 perfect feet scrub recipes for you:

15. Oaty Cornmeal Foot Scrub

Oats make great scrubs and when cornmeal is added to it, you will have feet that are squeaky clean!

Ingredients

½ cup oats

½ cup cornmeal

3 tbsp. sea salt

5 drops of lemon essential oil

2 drops eucalyptus essential oil

Process

Grind the oats to a powder in a food processor and then add cornmeal and salt to it. Mix well and then add the essential oils. Store in a glass jar. When using, take out ½ a cup of the scrub and mix with some lukewarm water. When a thick paste is formed, massage it into your feet. Rinse off with a wash cloth and then rinse with cool water.

16.   Get Rid of Smelly Feet Scrub

Are your feet always enclosed in sneakers or other closed shoes? Well then they must stink like anything! Try this scrub to get pretty-smelling feet.

Ingredients

2/3 cup of Epsom salt

1/3 cup of raw sugar

½ tbsp. dried peppermint

1 ½ tbsp. coconut oil

5 drops tea tree oil

5 drops peppermint oil

Process

Mix all the ingredients together and store in a glass jar. When you come home after a long day, wet your feet and rub this scrub on your feet. Massage for 2-3 minutes and then dip your feet for 10 minutes in a tub of hot water. Pat dry.

17.   Divine Scrub

This divine scrub will leave you yearning for more!

Ingredients

1 cup Epsom salt

½ cup grapeseed oil

2 tbsp. dried lavender buds

8-10 drops of lavender essential oil

A few drops of mint essential oil

Process

Combine all the ingredients together and store into a clean jar. Whenever you are about to take a bath, be sure to use this foot scrub first. Make sure you wash your feet with cold water.

18.   Bergamot Foot Scrub

Once you use this foot scrub, the heavenly smell and the sheer softness of your feet will never let you use anything else! Here is how you can make it:

Ingredients

½ cup raw sugar

½ cup coconut oil

½ cup sea salt

15 drops of bergamot essential oil

5 drops of sandalwood essential oil

Process

Simply combine all the ingredients together and store in a tightly-lidded jar. Whenever you are in the mood to give yourself a home pedicure, simply take out this scrub and massage it onto your feet. Wash off with warm water and pat dry.

19. Strawberry for the Feet

Ingredients

8-10 fresh strawberries

3 tbsp. sea salt or white granulated sugar

2 tbsp. sweet almond oil

Few drops of lemon essential oil

Process

Mash the strawberries in the rest of the ingredients. Store in a glass jar and massage on the foot whenever in the mood for luxury. Wash off with cool water and see the effects.

5 Scalp Scrubs

Shampoo may not be enough to clean your scalp and hair. If you want to make sure that no residues are left and your hair is squeaky clean, try using these scrubs and see how your hair starts to shine.

20. Lemon and Nut Scrub

This nutty and lemony scrub will leave your scalp clean and your hair pretty.

Ingredients

4 tbsp. coconut oil

2 tbsp. cane sugar

A few drops of lemon juice

Process

All you need to do is mix the ingredients and apply to hair. Massage gently for 2 minutes and leave in hair for 10 more minutes. Wash off with shampoo; make sure you give your scalp a cold water rinse at the end.

21.   Sugary Tea Tree Scrub

Brown sugar is a wonder for your whole external body. Use it on the scalp to see its wonderful results.

Ingredients

2 tbsp. raw brown sugar

5 drops of tea tree oil

5 tbsp. jojoba oil

A few drops of mint essential oil

Process

Mix all the ingredients and massage softly into hair for 2 minutes. Once done, wash off with cool water. Try using this every week to see excellent results.

22.   Egg Scrub

Eggs are perhaps the best products you can use for your hair. Mix them with olive oil and you get something that is unrivalled!

Ingredients

1 whole egg

2 tbsp. olive oil

1 tbsp. apple cider vinegar

1 tsp. fenugreek seeds

A few drops of lavender essential oil

Process

Mix all the ingredients together and apply to hair. Massage for 3 minutes, then cover your head and leave for 30 minutes. Wash off with warm water and then give your head a cool water rinse. You will notice a difference immediately.

23.   Honey scrub

This honey scrub may seem like a sticky toffee and, trust us, it will smell just as good, but it is excellent for your scalp and hair.

Ingredients

½ cup raw honey

1 cup white or brown sugar

1 tbsp. white vinegar

A few drops of rosemary essential oil

Process

Combine all the ingredients and apply to hair. Massage gently and leave on for 10 minutes. Wash off thoroughly. Once you are done be sure to give your hair a cold water rinse.

24.   Salty Scrub

Even though most of the scrubs for scalp mentioned here are sweet, this salty scrub can give the others a run for their money. Try it before assuming it won't work.

Ingredients

5 tbsp. Epsom salt

1 tbsp. white granulated sugar

3 tbsp. olive oil

A few drops of rose essential oil

Process

Mix the ingredients, apply to hair and massage gently for a minute or two. Let sit in hair for 5-10 minutes and then wash off with warm water. Do not forget to give your hair a cold water rinse at the end.

25 Effective Masks

If you feel that scrubs are enough to make your body and face soft and supple, then you are wrong. Scrubs remove the dead cells and skin–masks are the ones who nourish the skin and provide the shine and softness you desire. Here are some easy recipes for you to follow. Make sure that you try them on a small patch of skin before using them elsewhere.

Also keep in mind that using the masks once may not be enough. You will have to add it to your regular skin care routine to see some improved effects.

5 Body Masks

The body masks given below are not only easy, they are also very effective. As soon as you start using them, you will notice a significant change in the way you look and feel. Try each one out to see what works best for you.

25.　　Apple Pie for Body

Sounds delicious? It is! But please don't eat it, as it is to beautify your body. Try applying it at least once a week and see the results.

Ingredients

2 tbsp. fresh apple puree

4 tbsp. brown sugar

4 tbsp. white granulated sugar

A pinch of cinnamon

2 tbsp. sweet almond oil

A few drops of apple essential oil

Process

Combine all the ingredients and mix well. Just before bath, apply the mask to a slightly damp skin and rub in circular motions using a loofah. Wash off with warm water and then apply lotion. Your skin will smell divine!

26.   Chocolaty Delight!

Do you love chocolate? How about dark chocolate? Not only is it rich in antioxidants, it is also great for dry skin as a moisturizer. Try this spa luxury bathing mask and see how it feels!

Ingredients

½ cup milk

½ cup crushed dark chocolate

A few drops of tea tree essential oil

Process

Heat up the milk and add chocolate to it. Cook until all the chocolate is well combined, forming chocolate milk. You only have to use half this mixture for the bath. The rest can be stored in the fridge for 4 days. Once the chocolate milk is done, prepare a warm bath and add the milk and essential oil to it. Lay down in the bath for as long as you like and then rinse off with clean water.

27.   Avocado Mask

Avocados are amazing and can make your body so soft and glowing. Try this mask and see the results yourself.

Ingredients

2 ripe avocados, crushed

1 tbsp. almond oil

½ cup sea salt

1 tsp. lemon juice

A few drops of lime essential oil

Process

Mix together all the ingredients and cover your whole body with it. Let it sit on for about 15-20 minutes and then wash off with warm water. Apply lotion and see how you feel!

28.   Pumpkin Mask

Pumpkins don't only make yummy pies, they also create some wonderful body masks. Try this one to see if you like it as much as your pie!

Ingredients

½ cup pumpkin puree

1 tbsp. honey

1 tbsp. coconut oil

2 tbsp. bentonite clay

2 tsp. cinnamon

A few drops of lavender essential oil

Process

Mix ingredients, apply to body and leave on for 10 minutes. Wash off and you will immediately notice how silky smooth your skin gets. Have fun!

29.   Soothing Mask

When you are tired from a week of extensive work, this bath mask will help you shed off all the stress and anxiety.

Ingredients

½ cup baking soda

2 tbsp. white granulated sugar

A pinch of cloves, grounded

½ tsp. of ginger, grounded

1 tsp. cinnamon, grounded

A handful of fresh mint leaves

Process

Combine all the ingredients and store them in a glass jar. You can keep this bath mixture in the fridge and use it whenever you feel like relaxing in the bath. All you have to do is take about 2 tbsp. of the mixture and mix it in a hot water bath,then luxuriate.

5 Face Masks

Like the rest of your body, you need to pamper your face as well. These masks will make sure that they take all the strain away and leave you with a fresh and rejuvenated face. Try them all.

30. Yogurt Oatmeal Mask

This oatmeal mask will clean away all the dirt and dead cells. Try it today and see.

Ingredients

1 cup oatmeal, finely grounded

1 tsp. tightly-packed brown sugar

1 egg white

2 tbsp. yogurt

1 tsp. sweet almond oil

Process

Mix all the ingredients together and form a paste. Apply this to face and leave on for 10 minutes. Then rub lightly and wash off with tap water.

31.   Pineapple Exfoliating Mask

Pineapple has amazing clarifying properties. Mix it with papaya and you have something that will leave your face clear and shiny.

Ingredients

¼ cup fresh pineapple, cubed

¼ cup papaya, cubed

1 tbsp. honey

1 tsp. brown sugar

1 tbsp. almond oil

Process

Combine both the fruits and mash them well, so that they become soft and pulpy. Add all the other ingredients to the mush and apply to face. Leave on for 6-8 minutes and then wash off.

32.   Anti-Aging Mask

Avocados are great for you, be it your internal organs, hair or body. For the face, they help in keeping the skin hydrated and young looking. Here is how you can make the mask.

Ingredients

½ avocado

1 peeled carrot

1 egg yolk

1 tbsp. honey

1 tsp. lemon juice

½ tbsp. coconut oil

Process

Boil the carrot so it gets soft, and then mash them in the blender with avocados. Add in all the other ingredients and apply to face and neck. Leave on for 15 minutes. Wash off with a cloth soaked in warm water and then rinse the face with cool water.

33.   Aloe Vera Wonder

Aloe is perhaps one of the most effective treatments for all kinds of skin conditions. Try this mask and if you are not allergic, you will have something you won't ever want to leave.

Ingredients

2 tbsp. fresh aloe vera pulp

1½ tbsp. dry oatmeal

½ ripe avocado, mashed well

1 tsp. almond oil

1 tbsp. honey, warm in oven so it's runny

Process

Mix all the ingredients together and form a paste. Apply on clean face and leave on for 10-15 minutes. Wash off with warm water and see the shine!

34. Strawberry Delight

Strawberries have great anti-oxidizing properties, which mean they are wonderful for face uplifting and revitalized skin.

Ingredients

¼ cup fresh strawberries

¼ cup yogurt

A few drops of lavender essential oil

Process

Blend yogurt and strawberries in a blender so that they form a smooth paste. Add the essential oil and apply to face. Leave on for 10 minutes and wash off with tap water. Rinse with cold water and feel beautiful.

5 Hand Masks

Hands are that part of your body that are most used and become easily ragged. This is the reason you need to pay special attention to them so that they remain beautiful and young forever. These recipes will help you do just that.

35.   Potato Goodness

Potatoes are known for their rejuvenating properties. Add some milk to them and you will have the perfect hand softening recipe.

Ingredients

2 potatoes

Milk as per need

1 tbsp. sweet almond oil

A few drops of mint essential oil

Process

Boil the potatoes, mash them mix in milk and oils and apply the mixture on hands. Remove when the mixture cools down. Wash hands thoroughly. Do this at least once every week for soft supple hands.

36. Olive Castor Concoction

Olive oil and castor oil are both great softeners that make sure that the skin hydrated and elastic. Try this soak and see for yourself.

Ingredients

3 tbsp. olive oil

3 tbsp. castor oil

1 tsp. lemon juice

2 drops of lavender essential oil

Process

Mix the two base oils and warm them up a little. Add the lemon juice and lavender essential oil and soak your hands in the mixture for 15-20 minutes. After 10 minutes, massage the oil on your hands and let soak for another 5-10 minutes. Wash off the oil and pat dry.

37.   Avocado Mask

As mentioned earlier, avocados are great for skin conditioning, be it hands or face. Try this mask for both your hands and feet.

Ingredients

1 ripe avocado, mashed

2 tbsp. honey

2 tbsp. yogurt

10 drops sandalwood

8 drops myrrh

1 tbsp. olive oil

Process

Process all the ingredients in the blender and apply to hands. Wrap a plastic bag around the hands so that the mixture soaks in completely. Let sit for 15 minutes and then wash off.

38.   Egg Hand Mask

Do not worry about the smell, try the mask and you will soon forget the bad odor of the mask.

Ingredients

1 egg yolk

1 tbsp. lemon juice

1 tbsp. olive oil

Process

Beat the egg, oil and lemon juice together, for as long as it takes the mixture to get creamy. Then put your hands in it and coat completely. Wait for 15-20 minutes and then wash off.

39. Dry Hands Mask

If you suffer from dry hands, then this mask will make your hands conditioned and well nourished.

Ingredients

¼ cup brown sugar

2 tbsp. cranberry juice

A few drops of peppermint essential oil

Process

Mix all the ingredients and rub it on your hands. Leave on for 10 minutes and wash off with warm water. Then rinse with cool water.

5 Feet Masks

Just like your hands, your feet also get beaten up, which means you need to take extra care to make them look happy and healthy. Try these masks on a regular basis and you will notice a visible difference.

40.   Buttermilk Mask

Buttermilk is an excellent remedy for dry and dull looking feet. This mask is sure to give your feet a refreshed look.

Ingredients

1/3 cup rolled oats

1 cup buttermilk

1 capsule of vitamin A

A few drops of rosemary essential oil

Process

Add oaks to buttermilk and soak for a few hours. Strain and add vitamin A and essential oil. Mix and apply to feet. Wait for 15 minutes and then rinse off.

41.   Honeyed Yogurt Mask

The goodness of honey and yogurt is well known and, when applied to tired feet, it will leave them sparkly clean within no time.

Ingredients

1 egg yolk

3 tbsp. yogurt

2 tbsp. honey

1 tsp. Vitamin A

Few drops of grapefruit essential oil

Process

Mix all the ingredients together and apply to clean feet. Wash off after 15 minutes and you will feel like you just got back from a pedicure.

42. Cracked Feet Mask

If you have been suffering from cracked heels for a very long time, this mask will work wonders for you. All you need to do is use it at least once each week. Here is how you can make it:

Ingredients

4 tbsp. ground rice

2 tbsp. honey

1-2 tbsp. apple cider vinegar

1 tsp. olive oil

Process

Mix all the ingredients together and apply the paste to the cracked heels. Leave on for 20 minutes and then wipe off with a cloth soaked in warm water. Once clean, rinse your feet with cold water.

43. Milk Powder Mask

Milk powder can work wonders for your dry and peeling cracked heels. Try this mask and getting the dead skin off will be no problem.

Ingredients

5 tbsp. milk powder

2 tbsp. honey

2 tbsp. olive oil

10 drops of lavender essential oil

Process

Mix all the ingredients together and apply the mask to cracked heels. Leave on for 10 minutes, then gently rub your feet and wash off with warm water. Be sure to rinse with cold water at the end.

44.   Spicy Foot Treatment

Try this spicy treatment at home and watch your feet transform within 10 minutes.

Ingredients

4 tbsp. white sugar, grinded

1 tsp. cinnamon

A pinch of nutmeg

A pinch of cardamom

¼ cup papaya, mashed

A few drops of your favorite essential oil

2 tbsp. coconut oil

Process

Mix together all the ingredients and apply the mixture to feet. Rub in circular motion and then leave on for 10 minutes. Wash off with warm water and pat dry.

5 Hair Masks

Your hair should not be ignored. Like the rest of the body, they too need nourishment and special attention. By using scrubs and masks on your hair, you allow them to shed the dead skin, hair and any other buildup. Try using all these masks and see results.

45. Banana Egg Mask

Banana and eggs are both great for the scalp. Try using them and you will see that, not only does your hair get more soft and shiny, dandruff disappears too.

Ingredients

1 egg

1 ripe banana, mashed

1 tsp. sweet almond oil

A few drops of lime essential oil

Process

Mix all the ingredients together, so that a paste is formed. Apply to slightly wet hair and cover with a plastic bag. Wash off with tap water. Be sure to rinse thoroughly.

46.   Mayo Strawberry Mask

Mayo and strawberries are excellent for dry hair. They provide the right nourishment and keep the hair hydrated.

Ingredients

3 tbsp. mayonnaise

3 mashed strawberries

1 tsp. of coconut oil

A few drops of grapefruit essential oil

Process

Mix all the ingredients well and apply to slightly wet hair. Let the mask sit for about 30 minutes or so and then wash off. Be sure to rinse well.

47.   Rum Tea Mask

Sounds weird? It is excellent for your hair. Try using it to see how it works for your hair.

Ingredients

2 tsp. rum

2 tsp. cooked tea

A few drops of tea tree essential oil

Process

Combine all the ingredients and apply to the roots of your hair. Leave on for 50 minutes and then wash off. You will notice that your hair starts getting stronger.

48. Milk Honey Mask

Honey and milk are both great to consume as well as to put in hair. Try this mask and see the results.

Ingredients

5 tbsp. milk

2 tbsp. honey

1 tsp. rosewater

A few drops of lavender essential oil

1 tsp. of brown sugar

Process

Mix all the ingredients together and apply to wet hair. Cover with a warm towel and leave on for 45 minutes. Wash thoroughly afterwards. Your hair will become all silky smooth.

49. Avocado Lemon Mask

Avocados and lemons are both amazing for your hair. Try using this mask every other week. Keep in mind though that regular use of lemon will lighten the color of your hair.

Ingredients

½ ripe avocado, mashed

2 tbsp. lemon juice

1 tbsp. sweet almond oil

1 egg

A few drops of your favorite essential oil

Process

Combine all the ingredients together and apply to slightly wet hair. Leave on for an hour and then wash off. Be sure to shampoo. Your hair will become so beautiful you won't be able to keep your hands off it!

Conclusion

And there you have all the wonderful scrubs and masks recipes! Be sure to try as many as you can, but do be careful not to use anything that you might be allergic to. The great thing about these homemade formulas is that you can use them for yourself or gift wrap and present them to your loved ones. Have fun exploring the possibilities!

www.ingramcontent.com/pod-product-compliance
Lightning Source LLC
Chambersburg PA
CBHW081859280526
45789CB00007B/2767